Baby Food: Essential Guide for Supermoms

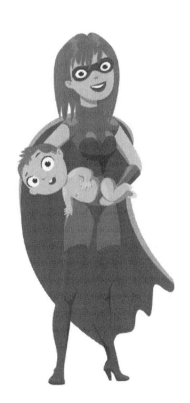

Disclaimer and Terms of Use: Effort has been made to ensure that the information in this book is accurate and complete, however, the author and the publisher do not warrant the accuracy of the information, text and graphics contained within the book due to the rapidly changing nature of science, research, known and unknown facts and internet. The Author and the publisher do not hold any responsibility for errors, omissions or contrary interpretation of the subject matter herein. This book is presented solely for motivational and informational purposes only.

Contents

Introduction

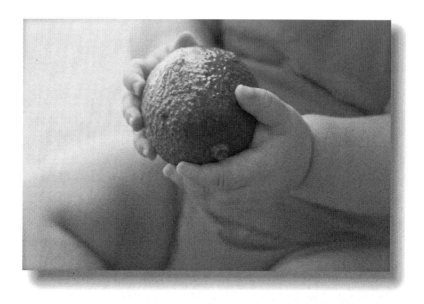

Hello, Supermoms! Welcome to your Essential Guide to Baby Food.

It's an exciting first step when your little one starts to move towards joining the world of fine dining and exotic tastes. One day, your bundle of joy will be enjoying pizza with friends after school, crab legs and canapes at their favorite restaurant, and fine wine with a significant other. But first, they have to conquer the basics of Baby Food — and so do you!

Moving your child from a liquid diet of breastmilk or formula to progressively more solid foods is not always as simple as it may sound. Many mothers find feeding baby to be one of the more daunting and cumbersome tasks of the first year. However, with this easy-to-follow guide at your fingertips, you can teach your baby to eat with confidence and skill. With the right knowledge in hand, you will minimize headaches and ensure that your baby develops his or her eating skills quickly, efficiently, and as enjoyably as possible.

We'll be covering the basics of how to safely introduce your little one to solids, and how to avoid common roadblocks to baby food success. We've even put together 25 Baby Food Recipes for easy reference when you want to pull together a nutritious and delicious meal for your growing baby.

The transition from liquids to solids is no easy task. There are many facets to consider, including:

- When to introduce solid foods?
- What is the difference between a puree and a mash, and when to use them?
- How to best prepare baby foods
- How to avoid constipation, messes, and other common problems
- Which is better, homemade or store bought?
- Which foods should come first?
- How can I make feeding time fun?
- How will my baby's feeding regimen change from birth to three years?
- What about allergies?
- What mistakes should I watch out for?
- How can I make delicious, awesome-tasting baby food?

This Guide will give you the answers to all of these questions and more. As we move forward, keep in mind that every baby is different, and what works for one may not work for another. Thus, this book is truly meant as a 'guide' rather than a prescriptive approach. Don't be afraid to experiment to find the best way to meet your baby's needs. Always consult your doctor if in doubt or before implementing a new developmental regimen, including baby feeding.

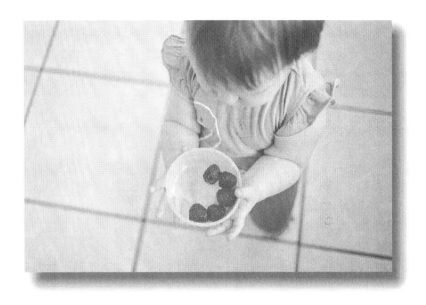

There are a number of different approaches for introducing your baby to solid foods. They each have their own strengths and weaknesses, with firm advocates and detractors on either side. The tips and tricks included in this guide draw from the best of two of the most popular approaches. Let's take a quick look at some different perspectives on this important milestone in your baby's life.

The Traditional Approach: Spoon Feeding and Purees

For many years, starting with purees and spoon feeding them to your baby was the norm, and today, many parents still prefer this method. If you're most comfortable with an old-school approach that worked for your mother and grandmother, this might be the way to go.

This method is all about giving your baby a gradual, gentle introduction to the world of solid foods. Beginning between four and six months, mothers start feeding their babies pureed foods mixed with breastmilk or formula.

New, progressively more solid foods are introduced slowly over time. Babies are usually fed on a set schedule. Mom or another caretaker 'spoons' the food into the baby's mouth for them, until they are old enough to begin doing it themselves.

Baby Led Weaning (BLW)

Baby Led Weaning, or BLW, is all about letting your baby be in control of his or her eating. Rather than trying to spoon feed your baby and force them to eat when and what you want them to, you simply give them options and guide them in feeding themselves.

BLW begins between six and eight months of age. This method advocates that you never put food in the baby's mouth, although you may help guide their hand towards their mouths to teach them to do it themselves. Rather than starting with purees, BLW starts with 'table foods,' regular solid foods that have been softened, mashed, and/or cut to help baby safely eat and digest them.

The following table sums up the differences between these methods:

	Spoon Feeding Method	Baby Led Weaning
Begin:	• 4-6 months	• 6-8 months
Method:	• Begin with purees diluted with breastmilk or formula and work up to increasingly solid foods and greater baby independence	• Begin with table foods and give baby control and independence from the beginning
Foods:	• Pureed and mashed vegetables, fruits, cereals, meats, and mixes • Focus on 'baby' foods designed just for babies	• Softened and/or mashed whole foods • Focus on 'real' foods being eaten by the rest of the family
Benefits:	• Gradual, gentle transition to progressively more solid foods	• Baby is in control of his or her own eating • Often starts later, so baby's digestive system is more developed • Less time spent prepping
Risks and Problems:	• Feeding too early may	• Messy • Possible

	<ul><li>cause allergies</li><li>Baby is less independent</li><li>Possibly linked to later obesity in some children</li></ul>	<ul><li>increase in choking risk</li><li>Potentially less nutritious as baby is in control of what he/she eats</li></ul>
Tips:	<ul><li>In the beginning, mix baby food purees with breastmilk or formula to ease the transition of both taste and texture</li><li>Start with an easy-to-digest, gluten-free grain such as rice porridge</li></ul>	<ul><li>Even though baby is eating independently, always monitor during feeding time in case of choking</li><li>Don't push baby to eat; let them decide if they're full, hungry, or in the mood</li></ul>

1: Is It Time?

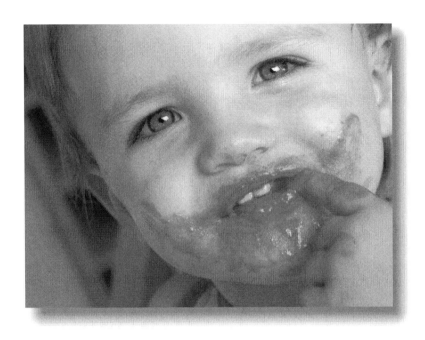

It's important to wait until your baby is ready before beginning the transition to solid foods. Beginning too early can result in digestive problems, allergies, increased risk of choking, and frustration for mom and baby alike. On the other hand, there's usually no reason to delay this important milestone if baby is ready to move on from a primarily liquid diet.

So how do you know when your baby is truly ready to join the world of solid food?

First of all, there are some important numbers to keep in mind. The CDC and the AAP both recommend that babies not be introduced to solid foods until six months or later. A number of studies have suggested that babies' digestive systems are not ready to process solid foods before this age, and beginning before six months can potentially lead to digestive problems and discomfort.

Introducing baby food too early can also increase the risk of your little one developing a food allergy.

On the other hand, for years pediatricians recommended introducing foods between four and six months of age, and a large number of doctors still make this recommendation today. Many parents have found success introducing food before six months, and some babies do seem to be ready earlier than others. Earlier than four months is not recommended.

Generally speaking, we agree with the CDC's recommendation of six months later. There is nothing to be lost by waiting a couple of extra months for your baby's digestive system to mature, and there is enough evidence correlating early weaning with food allergies to make the wait worth it.

With that in mind, how do you know when your baby is ready to start the journey towards solid food? There are a number of cues to keep in mind, most of which will come from your baby herself!

Start by noticing how your baby acts at meal time. You may notice him watching you with interest while you eat, mimicking mouth and tongue motions, or even smacking his lips. Being interested in food is a good sign that your baby is ready to start eating food.

All babies are born with a tongue thrust reflex. This reflex helps keep babies safe by pushing foreign objects (including food) out of their mouths. They will begin to lose it between four and six months of age, and it's usually disappeared by six months. The tongue thrust reflex should be gone before you start introducing foods.

If you think your baby is ready for solid foods, try giving them a little cereal. If it stays in their mouth (if they don't push it out with their tongue), they're probably ready.

For baby led weaning, your baby should also be able to sit up without help or support, hold her own head steady, and pick up her own food. It's okay if you need to guide their hands towards their mouths in the beginning, but they should be capable of putting the food in themselves.

2: 10 Tips for First Foods

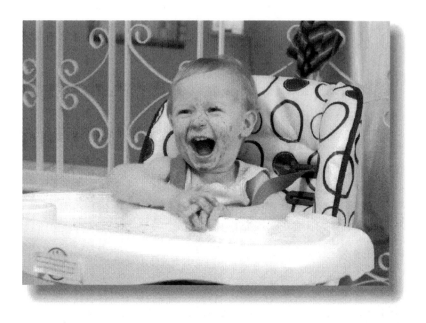

If your baby is ready to get started, it's time to move on to the first step: Introducing first foods! We've put together 10 easy rules to guide you as move forward. Keep in mind that these tips are not meant to be hard and fast 'prescriptions'; rather, use them as guidelines to inform your baby's personal journey and keep her on track for a healthy transition to eating.

Tip 1: Rice is often recommended as a first food because it is gluten-free and easy to digest. Pureed vegetables are another excellent introductory food that provide important nutrients. For BLW, avocados, sweet potatoes, and bananas are great first choices because they are gentle and easy to finger. The AAP recommends introducing your baby to a wide variety of healthy foods, in terms of both flavor and texture.

Tip 2: Try mixing your first baby purees with breastmilk or formula. Gradually increase the amount of puree or mash until your baby is eating at a regular consistency.

Tip 3: Start small. Try a tablespoon the first day and then gradually work up to more.

Tip 4: The first time you feed your baby food, don't try to replace his meal. Go ahead and feed him about half of his regular breastmilk or formula serving, or wait until an hour after he's eaten. The first attempt at baby food won't get it all down, and if your baby is hungry you will only cause frustration and discomfort.

Tip 5: Don't introduce new foods all at once. Wait 4 days before giving your baby her next food. This will allow you to watch for any allergies, and pinpoint what caused them if they develop.

Tip 6: Don't feed your baby directly from the container unless you're sure he will be able to finish it. To avoid contaminating leftovers with bacteria from your baby's mouth, scoop the baby food into its own serving dish. You can always add more if your baby is still hungry!

Tip 7: Watch out for choking—always monitor your baby during feeding, even if she is feeding herself. Chocking is a real hazard for babies, so be prepared to intervene if necessary.

Tip 8: Don't force your baby to eat. If he is refusing food, move on and try again later.

Tip 9: Your baby's brain needs healthy fats for proper development. Make sure to include baby-friendly servings of healthy fat sources, such as olive oil or avocados, in your baby's new diet.

Tip 10: If your baby doesn't seem to like a food, don't give up. It can take up to 10 exposures before a baby gets 'used' to a new taste and texture. In some cases, they may never develop a taste for those mashed peas, but much of the time they'll be happily gumming away after a few more chances to try things out.

3: Baby's First Foods

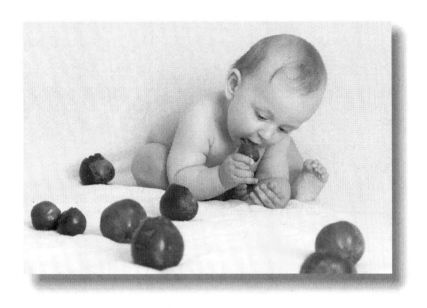

Which foods you choose to introduce your baby to first will depend on how old your baby is and which feeding method you've chosen to follow. Many health organizations, including the AAP, recommend that infants receive a variety of healthy, nutritious foods to complement breast milk or formula after 6 months. Which foods you choose will be largely up to you and your baby.

Generally speaking, if your baby is around six months and you choose the spoon-fed method, you'll probably be starting with baby cereals and porridges before moving on to pureed or mashed vegetables, fruits, and finally meats and dairy.

Many experienced mothers recommend fruits after vegetables because babies love the sweet taste of fruits and may be more resistant to vegetables once they know there's a sweeter option.

However, the truth is that babies like sweet foods; it's natural, and it will be true regardless of when fruits are introduced.

With baby fed weaning, you'll want to jump straight to table foods. Instead of delaying fruits, feel free to start with soft fruits such as mashed bananas, avocados, ripe melon, or pears or apples (steam first to soften). Mashed sweet potatoes and steamed butternut squash are another great choice for introducing your baby to solids.

If you choose to go all-out with the baby led weaning method, you should try to choose foods that your family is also eating. The aim is for the baby to join the real, authentic world of dinner and eating from the beginning, so avoid giving them separate food from the family.

This doesn't mean that if the rest of the family is eating tacos your baby is ready for a hard shell and sour cream. However, try to include some ingredients in the main meal that are baby-friendly and then give those to your baby. For example, give your baby avocado chunks and also put them on the table to go with your family's tacos. Give your baby a few options to choose from. Start with simple whole foods and work your way up to combinations and complexity.

Check out the following table for suggestions on what to introduce to your baby, and when. Please keep in mind that feeding from 4-6 months is not recommended for most babies. Make sure to check with your pediatrician before beginning a feeding program at this or any age. Always make sure that each of the following foods is soft enough and small enough for baby to swallow safely.

Age	Grains	Vegetables	Fruits	Meats	Dairy
4-6 months	Rice cereal	Pumpkin Carrots Sweet potato	Apple Avocado Banana Peach Pear	none	none
6-8 months	Barley cereal Oatmeal Wheat cereal	Bell pepper Broccoli Zucchini Butternut Squash	Apricot Kiwi Mango Melon Plums Prunes	Chicken Turkey	Yoghurt Cheese
8-10 months	Flax Millet Quinoa Buck wheat	Asparagus Beans Cauliflower Cucumber Eggplant Onions Parsnips	Blueberries Cherries Coconut Figs Persimmons Pineapple	Beef Eggs Lamb Pork	Same as before
10-12 months	Same as before	Corn Okra Spinach Tomatoes	Citrus Raspberries Strawberries	Fish	Cow's milk

19

4: Store-Bought vs Homemade

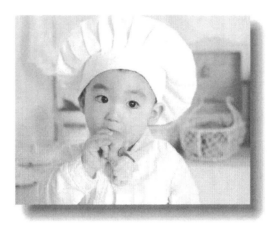

Whether to make your own baby food purees and mashes can be a tough choice. On the one hand, homemade food is usually more nutritious and free of preservatives. Homemade food lets you rest assured that you know what's in your baby's food and where it came from.

On the other hand, busy moms don't always have time to make baby food for every meal. Even making baby food in advance and freezing it won't always be practical. Further, homemade baby food doesn't keep as long, nor is it as portable. Store bought food can make life easier in many ways, by reducing the time you spend in the kitchen. It's also easy to pop into a diaper bag when you're on the go and don't want to worry about spoilage.

In the end, you'll probably use both at one time or another. As with adults, organic, seasonal fruits and vegetables are always the best choice.

Try to select seasonal fruits and vegetables when preparing food for your baby. If it's the wrong season for the food you had in mind, consider trying a different recipe. If you must buy fruits and vegetables out of season, try to choose organic foods to reduce your baby's exposure to pesticides.

We recommend making your baby food whenever possible, but if you do purchase baby food, rest assured that there are many good options on the market. While it's true that store-bought baby foods lose some nutrients due to the canning process, they still retain many essential vitamins and minerals for your baby. Many store-bought baby foods also have no added salts, sugars, or preservatives, so the food is natural and gentle for baby's tummy. Just remember to read labels to make sure.

When it comes to cooking, there are a few tips to keep in mind:

- Peel fruits and vegetables first
- Steam veggies rather than boil, as boiling depletes more nutrients
- Puree using a food processor or blender
- Save time by making larger batches and freezing them
- Freezing pureed baby food in an ice cube tray will give perfect baby-size portions for later use; cover the tray to keep it sanitary and pop the cubes into a freezer bag once they're frozen
- Add juices rather than sugar if you want to sweeten the recipe

Finally, keep in mind that some vegetables are not suited for home cooking with very young babies, because too many nitrates can get leeched into the water during preparation. While your baby is in early infancy, it's best that carrots, green beans, beets, and squash be purchased rather than prepared, as manufacturers are better able to test for nitrates.

For some easy, delicious baby food recipes, check out the 25 Baby Food Recipes included in this book.

5: Make Eating Fun!

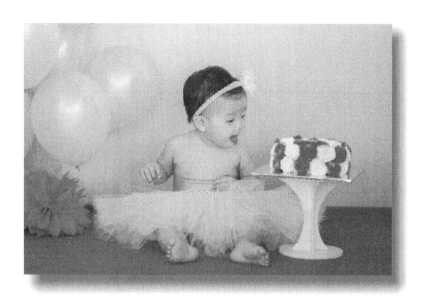

Many mothers—and babies—experience frustration when it comes to feeding time. From messes to distractions to refusal, weaning your baby onto solid foods can be a challenge.

Luckily, there many ways to make eating more fun! Learning to eat is a special time in your baby's life, one which will set the stage for their life-long relationship with food. Reducing frustration for you and your baby will let you more fully enjoy every moment as you watch your baby experience new tastes and sensations.

In the beginning, your baby will be interested (even fascinated) by the new sensations associated with eating and tasting. However, all too quickly they may lose interest in their new activity. At this point, distraction sets in and getting them to hold still for feeding time or try new foods becomes more difficult.

One solution to this problem is to stick to the baby led weaning method. Because BLW leaves your infant in charge of her own eating, you rarely have to struggle to get them to eat—if they don't want to, you simply move on and try again later.

However, regardless of method there will be times when you need your baby to eat a certain amount at a certain time. Try the following tips to make mealtime more enjoyable for everyone:

1: Don't be afraid of the messes! Rather than try to make your baby eat without making a mess, accept that messiness is part of the process. Have a system in place for quick and easy cleanup, and be proud of your baby's involvement in her own eating.

Tip 2: If you are spoon feeding your baby, let them hold the spoon as soon as they are able. Babies love to grasp and try things themselves, so letting them hold the spoon will keep their attention focused on the task at hand. They will also learn to feed themselves faster if you let them get involved in the feeding process.

Tip 3: Consider trying a loadable spoon. Just fill the dispenser and press a button to get a perfectly baby-sized spoonful every time your baby is ready for another bite. These will help minimize messes and are super convenient when you are out at the park or grabbing a quick feeding session around town.

Tip 3: Don't worry about manners. Feeding your baby during the first twelve months is all about making a healthy transition to solid food. For your baby, it's also about exploration and having sensory experiences. Don't be afraid to let them to suck the puree right off of their fingers.

Tip 4: Use a high chair. A properly cared for high chair is sanitary and easier to clean up when the meal is over.

Highchairs can also reduce your frustration as they make it more difficult for the baby to wiggle away. Learning to eat away from mom's lap is also good for establishing future eating habits.

Tip 5: Try using Nibblers. Nibblers are suckable feeding devices that help to introduce your baby to new tastes while minimizing the risk of choking. These colorful tools have a baby-friendly handle with a safe net pouch at the end in which you can put everything from frozen berries to mashed banana. Your baby can hold the Nibbler himself and gnaw on the net to suck the food out. Many babies enjoy the gnawing action almost as much as the taste, and with frozen fruit or vegetables in the net, these can even help with teething.

6: When to Feed Baby

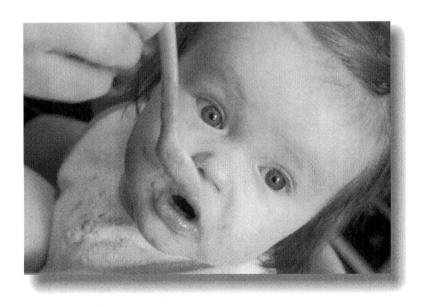

Babies have very tiny stomachs. Food moves through them quickly, so they need to eat far more often than older children or adults. How often and when your baby eats will change as they grow, especially once they're in the weaning stage, when they will be eating a combination of breastmilk or formula and solid foods.

In the early stages of introducing solids, the amount of baby food your baby eats should be determined by your baby. Baby food should not be your baby's primary source of nutrition until one year or later. Up until then, solid foods provide an important nutritional and experiential supplement to breastmilk and formula.

The following table will give you an idea of when, and how often, your baby should be eating based on age:

Age	Breastmilk / Formula	Solids
0-3 months	- 4-6 oz. per feeding - 6x/day - Every 2-3 hours	None
4-6 months	- 5-7 oz. per feeding - 5x/day - Every 4-5 hours	- None, or - 1x-2x per day
6-9 months	- 7-8 oz. per feeding - 4x/day - Every 4-6 hours	- 3x per day - At family mealtimes and designated snack time
9-12 months	- 7-8 oz. per feeding - 4x/day - Every 6 hours	- 3x-4x per day - At family mealtimes and designated snack time
12-18 months	- Continue if desired, allowing baby to self-regulate the amount - Include whole milk from 12 months	- 4x-6x per day - At family mealtimes and designated snack time
18-24 months	NA	- 4x-6x per day
24-36 months	NA	- 4x-6x per day

7: Baby Food and Allergies

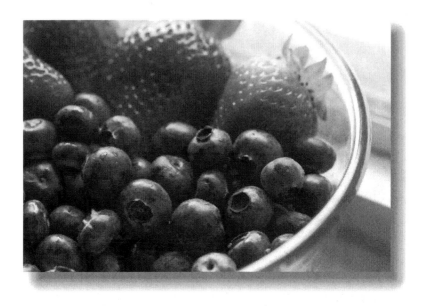

Food allergies can be a scary thing to encounter, with reactions ranging from the merely uncomfortable to the life threatening. If your baby is showing symptoms of an allergic reaction, it's imperative that you identify the food that's causing the allergy as early as possible, to avoid feeding it to your baby again.

In most cases, allergies will clear up once you've stopped feeding your baby the triggering food. However, if the reaction is severe, doesn't clear up in a day or two, or involves swelling or difficulty breathing, call your doctor or emergency services immediately. Even though most reactions won't be this severe, it's better to err on the side of safety, so when in doubt call your doctor.

To help you identify allergies as quickly as possible, many pediatricians recommend the 4 Day Rule. This means waiting four days after introducing one new food before introducing another. By limiting the introduction of new foods to just one at a time, you'll be able to quickly identify the culprit if an allergy pops up.

For example, if your baby suddenly starts sprouting hives, and the only new food in her diet was that cantaloupe you started giving her a few days ago, all you have to do is cut out the cantaloupe. If the hives go, chances are you've found the problem.

The chart below lists some of the most common allergy-causing foods for babies. Keep in mind that babies may develop an allergy to more than one food.

Most Common Allergens
Cow's milk
Eggs
Peanuts
Soy
Wheat
Tree nuts
Fish
Shellfish
Berries
Citrus Fruits
Tomatoes
Peas

Be especially attentive when introducing foods from the table above. Additionally, it is recommended that parents wait until about 1 year old to introduce strawberries, and 10 months for hard cheeses.

8: Healthy Habits

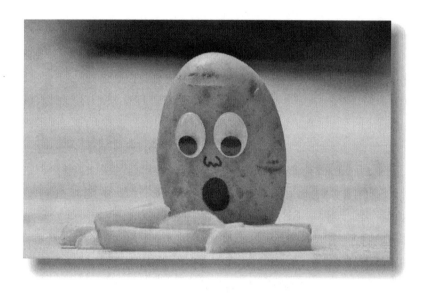

It's never too early to start building healthy habits into your baby's routine. Far too many children in today's world grow up overweight or obese and enter adulthood with an unhealthy, unsustainable relationship with food. Help your baby to avoid this fate by establishing healthy behaviors from the beginning.

Here are some things to remember when it comes to your baby's eating habits:

Food is Nourishment

To help your baby develop a healthy relationship with food, treat food as nourishment. Avoid using food as a reward, bribe, or distraction. Besides associating food with non-nourishment roles in your baby's mind, using food for these purposes can lead to a habit of asking for food when not hungry, eating for comfort, and overeating. All of these are prime ingredients for future weight problems.

Avoid Added Sugars and Salts

Natural, whole foods are usually the best option for all of us, and babies are no exception. Avoid adding too much sugar or salt to your baby's food unless directed to do so by a doctor. Too much sugar can lead to increased appetite, while salt is hard on babies' kidneys.

Instead, encourage your baby to develop a taste for healthy food by only sweetening food with natural fruit juices. Instead of adding salt, add variety of flavor by combining whole-foods ingredients, such as peas and roast beef.

Don't Eat in Front of the TV

Letting your baby eat while watching tv can lead to 'mindless' eating, or eating on autopilot. This will interfere with your baby's ability to recognize when they are full and can lead to overeating. Instead, try to provide a consistent time and place for feeding—preferably at the family table, when the family is eating—and teach baby to focus on and enjoy mealtimes.

Don't Forget the Fat

The low-fat craze left us all a bit wary of this macronutrient, but the truth is that the right fats in the right amounts are necessary for our bodies to be healthy. For your baby, fat is also imperative for healthy brain development. If you're only feeding your baby fruits and vegetables, you're depriving them of this vital nutrient. You'll need to make sure there are enough healthy sources of fat in their baby food, including avocados and olive oil. Your baby should develop a taste for all of the important nutrients that she will be eating throughout her life, including healthy fat. Talk to your doctor to determine just how much fat your baby needs.

Provide Structure

As your baby becomes older and more independent in making food choices, he will start to ask for foods more frequently, especially after 12 months of age. It can be tempting to give in to frequent requests for food, juice, or milk, but help your little one learn to self-regulate by sticking to a snack and mealtime schedule.

Have them eat at the table with the rest of the family, and set up consistent snack times for those extra bites that babies and toddlers need. This will help them learn to wait a developmentally appropriate space of time between feedings and avoid relying on food as entertainment.

9: Pitfalls to Avoid

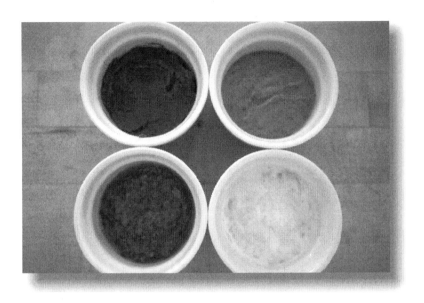

Making mistakes is a part of parenting that can't be avoided. When it comes to feeding your baby, the best way to avoid making mistakes is to be aware of potential pitfalls so that you can intervene before they get out of hand. Here are some common issues to watch out for.

Constipation

When you start towards more solid food, constipation can be an issue. In the beginning, your baby may only be eating diluted cereal that is mostly breastmilk. As you start diluting less, add some baby prunes or apples to one meal/day to help regulate your baby's system. The same holds true if you are going with the BLW method—make sure that they have high-fiber foods like baby prunes available as a food choice.

Weaning too Soon

Although you may start introducing solid foods around six months, you aren't actually weaning until you begin to reduce breastmilk or formula intake, eventually eliminating it completely.

Although it's exciting to see your baby become increasingly independent with her feeding, don't rely on solids for mealtime just yet. Although you may begin some reduction as early as six months if your baby is ready, whenever possible, breastmilk or formula should remain a steady part of your baby's diet until at least one year of age.

Starting too Early

As previously discussed, introducing solid foods too early can be detrimental to your baby's digestion and contribute to an increased risk for food allergies. To avoid these problems, only give your baby breastmilk or formula prior to four months. Consult your pediatrician and consider carefully before deciding to feed your baby before six months. For best results, begin introducing solid foods at six months or later.

Starting too Late

Although less common, sometimes parents wait too long to start introducing solid foods. Solid foods are an important part of your baby's growing nutritional needs, particularly in terms of fat and iron. The older your baby gets, the less that breastmilk and formula can cover the bases for these important brain-specific nutrients. If your baby isn't eating solid foods by eight months, consult your pediatrician to ensure that they are getting adequate nutrition.

Forcing Baby to Eat

Babies are naturally good at self-regulating their food intake. When a baby shakes his head, turns his face, or closes his mouth, it's okay to listen to these cues. Forcing your baby to keep eating after he is full can interfere with his ability to recognize satiety. If your baby seems full or disinterested in continuing the meal, try once or twice more and then stop. Letting your baby control whether they will eat will help them to build healthier food regulation habits.

10: 25 Easy Baby Food Recipes

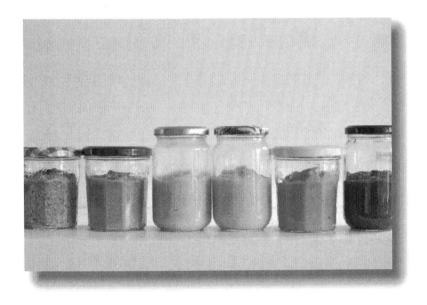

We promised 25 Easy Baby Food Recipes and here they are!

Keep this reference handy whenever you're ready to try out a new meal with your little one. All of these recipes can be batched and frozen to save you time in the kitchen. Just make sure that your baby has been introduced to each ingredient using the 4 Day Rule before trying a new recipe.

Bon Appétit!

Grains

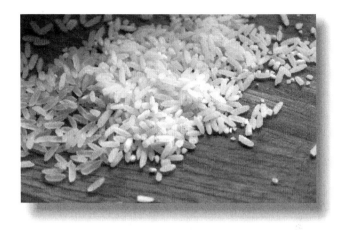

Rice Cereal

Ingredients

- ¼ cup rice powder
- 1 cup water

Directions

1. Bring the water to a boil.
2. While stirring, add the rice powder.
3. Simmer for about 10 minutes, stirring continuously.

Tip: You can make your own rice powder by grinding brown rice, or a blend of brown and white rice, in a food processor.

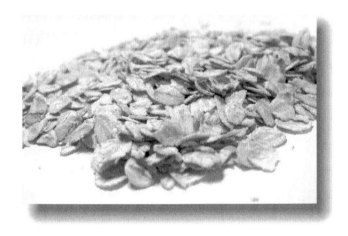

Oatmeal Cereal

Ingredients

- ¼ cup ground, steel-cut oats
- ¾ cup to 1 cup water

Directions

1. Bring the water to a boil.
2. While stirring, add the ground oats.
3. Simmer for 15-20 minutes, stirring frequently.

Tip: Although steel-cut oats take longer to cook, they retain more nutrients than instant or quick-cook oats.

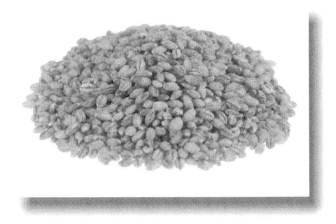

Barley Cereal

Ingredients

- ¼ cup ground barley
- 1 cup water

Directions

1.   Bring water to a boil.
2.   While stirring, add the barley.
3.   Simmer for 10 minutes, stirring constantly.

Tip: After cooking, stir in some breastmilk, formula, or juice for extra flavor and nutrition.

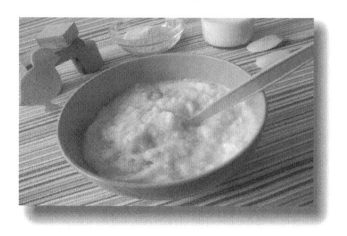

Fruity Rice Porridge

Ingredients

- ½ cup rice cereal
- ½ cup apple sauce
- ¼ cup white grape juice

Directions

1.   In a medium sauce pan, combine rice porridge and white grape juice
2.   Heat slowly, stirring constantly; do not allow to boil
3.   Stir in the applesauce

   Tip: Grape juice can be replaced with apple juice, pear juice, or even peach juice for a whole different flavor.

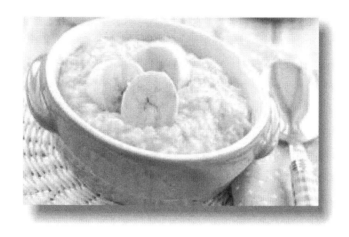

Banana Rice Bowl

Ingredients

- ½ cup rice cereal
- 1 ripe banana

Directions

1.   Mash banana with a fork
2.   Mash rice cereal into banana
3.   Mix until a smooth, even consistency is achieved

Tip: Serve at room temperature for best results.

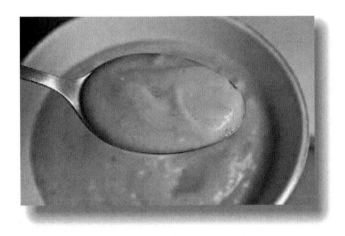

Apricot Puree

Ingredients

- 1 cup chopped apricots
- 1 cup apple juice, white grape juice, or water

Directions

1.   In a small-medium saucepan, bring fruit and liquid to a boil.
2.   Simmer for 8-10 minutes
3.   Strain the mixture into a blender; save the leftover liquid.
4.   Use the blender to puree the mixture. Add the leftover liquid until you achieve the desired consistency.

Tip: If your puree is too thin, try adding a little baby cereal to thicken it up.

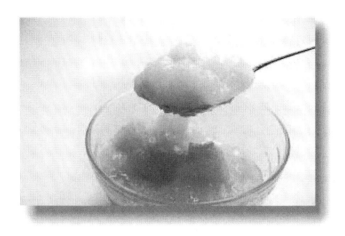

Mixed Fruit Applesauce

Ingredients

- 1 cup peeled apple chunks (make sure to completely remove the core)
- ½ cup fruit of your choice (recommended: berries or pears)
- 1 ½ cups water

Directions

1.   Add fruit and water to a medium saucepan.
2.   Boil until the fruit is tender.
3.   Drain, saving the leftover liquid.
4.   Mash fruit mixture using a fork or potato masher.
5.   Place mixture into blender or food processor and puree.
6.   Add leftover liquid until you achieve the desired consistency.

Tip: Experiment with the ratio of apples to other fruits.

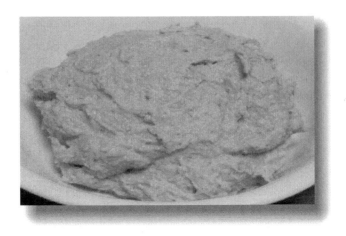

Banana Avocado Mush

Ingredients

- 1 ripe banana
- 1 ripe avocado

Directions

1.   Peel banana and add to a bowl.
2.   Peel avocado, remove seed and slice into chunks. Add to the bowl.
3.   Mash banana and avocado together with a fork until desired consistency is reached.

    Tip: Make sure the banana and avocado are both ripe to aid mashing and increase flavor.

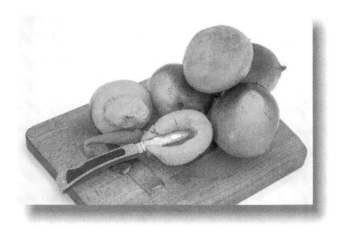

Mango Cubes

Ingredients

- 1 ripe mango

Directions

1. Peel mango and remove the seed
2. Cut the fruit into baby-sized chunks
3. Freeze

Tip: Make the mango chunks a little bigger than you might if adding to a food or salsa, so baby can hold them comfortably in one hand to gum or suck.

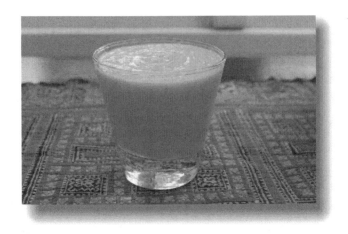

Peach Smoothie

Ingredients

- 1 ripe peach
- ~2 Tablespoons breastmilk or formula

Directions

1.   Steam the peach until soft
2.   Remove the skin and pit
3.   When cool, puree the fruit in a blender or food processor
4.   Add breastmilk or formula until desired consistency is achieved

Tip: Ask your pediatrician if it's okay to add a dash of cinnamon for fun and flavor.

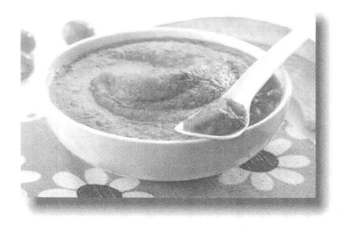

Mixed Veg

Ingredients

- ½ cup sliced carrots
- ½ cup chopped parsnips, peeled
- ½ cup frozen peas

Directions

1.   Steam carrots, peas, and parsnips until soft
2.   Drain
3.   Puree in a blender or food processor, adding extra water until desired consistency is achieved

Tips: Try cutting the parsnips into very small bite-sized pieces. Steam separately until very soft. Puree the carrots and peas and then stir in the parsnip pieces to give a baby a different texture and something to gum.

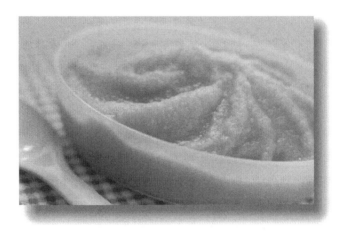

Dinner Veg

Ingredients

- ½ cup frozen green beans
- 1 peeled, cubed potato
- ½ cup zucchini
- ¼ cup chopped carrots

Directions

1.   Add all vegetables to a medium saucepan; cover with water to ½ inch above the surface of the vegetables.
2.   Boil until soft
3.   Mash with a fork or puree in a blender or food processor

    Tips: For added flavor, add a little low-sodium, all-natural chicken broth.

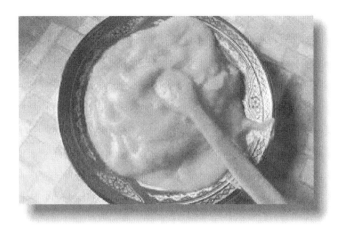

Squash Mix

Ingredients

- ½ cup chopped zucchini
- ½ cup chopped summer squash
- ½ cup peeled, chopped sweet potato
- 1 Tablespoon chopped onion

Directions

1.   Place vegetables in a medium saucepan; cover with water to ½ inch above the vegetables
2.   Simmer until soft
3.   Mash or puree until mix reaches desired consistency

Tip: When it comes to mixes, make sure that your baby has been previously introduced to each food used in the mix, using the 4 Day Rule to check for allergies.

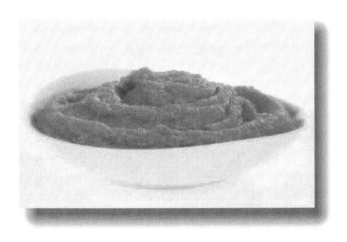

Berry Sweet Potatoes

Ingredients

- 1 sweet potato, peeled and cubed
- ½ cup frozen mixed berries, thawed (make sure baby has been introduced to each berry in the mix)

Directions

1. Steam the sweet potato cubes until soft
2. Drain, add to food processor or blender
3. Add thawed berries
4. Puree to desired consistency

Tip: Is it a fruit, or is it a vegetable? This mix gives baby the best of both worlds. Adjust the amount of berries to give your baby a different taste.

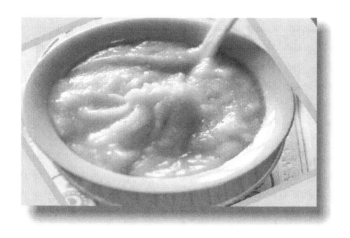

Cauliflower Mash

Ingredients

- 1 cup chopped cauliflower
- 1 cup frozen peas
- 1 cup baked butternut squash meat

Directions

1.   Steam frozen peas and chopped cauliflower until soft
2.   Add peas, cauliflower, and squash to a food processor or blender
3.   Puree to desired consistency

Tip: Saving ingredients from last night's dinner can save you time and headaches when it comes to making baby food. Try having butternut squash with the family the night before, and set some aside to use for purees the next day.

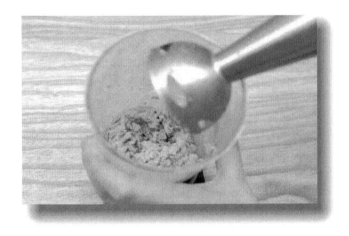

Basic Beef Puree

Ingredients

- 1 cup cubed, cooked beef
- ½ cup water

Directions

1. Add beef to a food processor or blender and create a fine puree
2. Continue to puree until desired consistency is achieved

Tip: Use this basic puree to create mixtures with your babies favorite pureed vegetables.

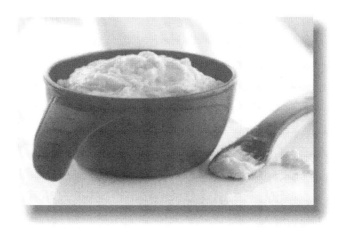

Basic Chicken Puree

Ingredients

- 1 cup cubed cooked chicken breast
- ½ cup low-sodium chicken broth

Directions

1.   Add beef to a food processor or blender and create a fine puree
2.   Continue to puree, adding broth until desired consistency is achieved

     Tip: When your baby is ready for dairy, try mixing this base with ½ cup yogurt for a different taste and texture.

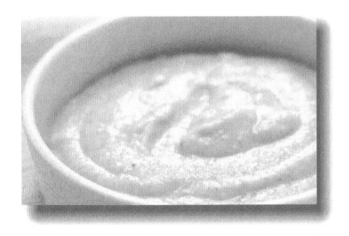

Basic Fish Puree

Ingredients

- 1 cup cooked boneless white fish
- ¼ cup water

Directions

1.   Add fish to food processor or blender
2.   Puree until desired consistency is reached, adding water as needed

Tip: Try adding some berries or apple sauce to this puree for added nutrition and a unique but delicious flavor.

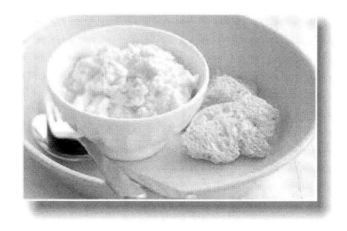

Baby Omelet

Ingredients

- 1 Egg Yolk
- ¼ cup milk
- ¼ cup shredded cheddar cheese
- ¼ cup pureed carrots

Directions

1. Combine ingredients in a bowl
2. Stir well
3. Add to skillet
4. Scramble until no longer runny

Tip: Try replacing the carrot puree with your baby's favorite vegetable for a whole new dish.

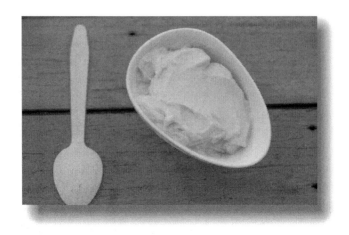

Creamy Chicken Casserole

Ingredients

- 1 chopped chicken breast
- 1 peeled and chopped potato
- ½ cup chopped carrots
- ½ cup chopped summer squash
- ½ cup yogurt

Directions

1.	Combine chicken, vegetables, and spices in a saucepan
2.	Cover with water and bring to a boil
3.	Reduce heat, cover, and simmer for 30-45 minutes or until chicken is fully cooked and vegetables are soft
4.	Let cool
5.	Add chicken and vegetables to food processor or blender and puree to desired consistency, adding left over liquid as needed
6.	Add yogurt, continue to puree to desired consistency

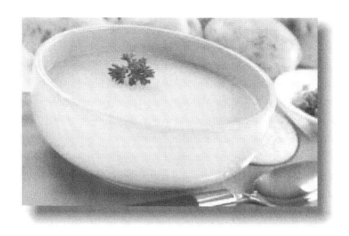

Chicken Soup

Ingredients

- 1 cup chopped chicken breast, uncooked
- ¼ cup chopped onion
- ¼ cup chopped carrot
- ½ cup chopped zucchini
- 4 cups water

Directions

1.   Combine ingredients in a saucepan and bring to a boil
2.   Reduce heat, cover, and simmer for 30-45 minutes, or until chicken is well cooked and carrots are soft
3.   Let cool
4.   Strain into to food processor or blender and puree, adding broth until desired consistency is reached

Tip: Try adding different vegetables, such as summer squash, peas, or cauliflower, for a different taste.

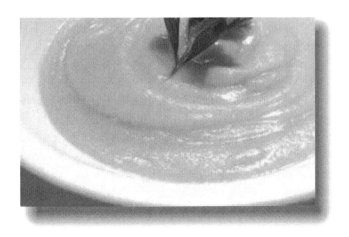

Vegetable Beef Soup

Ingredients

- 1 cup of chopped beef
- 1 peeled and chopped potato
- ½ cup chopped carrot
- ¼ cup chopped onion
- 5 cups water

Directions

1.   Place all ingredients in a saucepan and bring to a boil
2.   Reduce heat, cover, and simmer for 30-45 minutes or until beef is well cooked and vegetables are soft
3.   Let cool
4.   Add meat and vegetables to a food processor or blender and puree, adding broth until desired consistency is reached

Tip: Try using spices for varied taste.

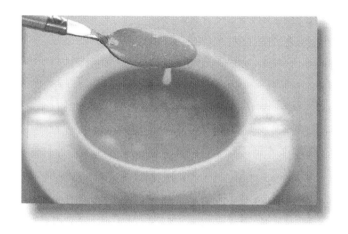

Pumpkin Soup

Ingredients

- 1 cup pumpkin puree
- 2 cups low-sodium chicken broth
- ¼ teaspoon black pepper
- ¼ teaspoon ginger
- 1 garlic clove, minced

Directions

1. Combine ingredients in a saucepan and bring to a boil
2. Reduce heat, cover, and simmer for 15 minutes, stirring often

Tip: Soups can be good cold, too! Try pouring this easy soup into an ice tray to make delicious frozen soup cubes.

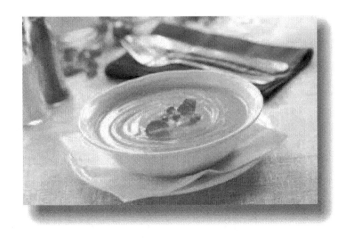

Butternut Squash Soup

Ingredients

- 1 cup steamed butternut squash meat
- ¼ cup steamed carrots
- 1/2 cup frozen spinach
- ½ cup frozen peas
- 2 cups low sodium chicken broth

Directions

1.   In a saucepan, bring all ingredients to a boil
2.   Reduce heat immediately
3.   Cover and simmer 10-15 minutes, stirring occasionally
4.   Let cool
5.   Add contents of saucepan to a food processor or blender and puree

Tip: Add yogurt for a creamier consistency.

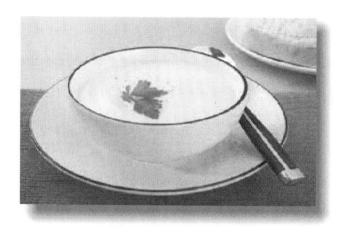

Egg Drop Soup

Ingredients

- 2 cups low sodium chicken broth
- 2 egg yolks
- diced cauliflower

Directions

1.   Bring chicken broth, cauliflower, and spices to boil in a saucepan

2.   Reduce heat, cover, and simmer 15-20 minutes or until cauliflower is soft

3.   While still simmering, stir in egg yolks with a wire whisk

4.   Continue whisking until egg yolk is solid

5.   Let cool

6.   Add to a food processor and puree

Tip: After adding the eggs and while still simmering, whisk in a little basic chicken puree for added protein.

89507418R00035

Made in the USA
Lexington, KY
29 May 2018